good morning yoga

yoga

a pose-by-pose wake up story

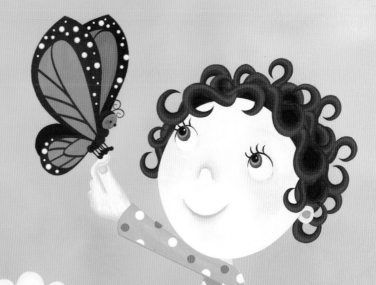

Mariam Gates

ILLUSTRATED BY
Sarah Jane Hinder

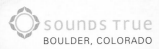
sounds true
BOULDER, COLORADO

Sounds True, Boulder, CO 80306

Copyright © 2016 Mariam Gates
Illustrations © 2016 Sarah Jane Hinder

Published 2016
Book design by Beth Skelley
Printed in South Korea

Names: Gates, Mariam, author. | Hinder, Sarah Jane, illustrator.
Title: Good morning yoga : a pose-by-pose wake up story / Mariam Gates ;
illustrated by Sarah Jane Hinder.
Description: Boulder, CO : Sounds True, 2016. | Audience: 4—8.
Identifiers: LCCN 2015037364 | ISBN 9781622036028
Subjects: LCSH: Hatha yoga for children—Juvenile literature.
Classification: LCC RJ133.7 .G39 2016 | DDC 613.7/046083—dc23
LC record available at http://lccn.loc.gov/2015037364

ISBN: 978-1-62203-602-8   Ebook ISBN: 978-1-62203-634-9

10 9 8 7 6 5 4 3 2 1

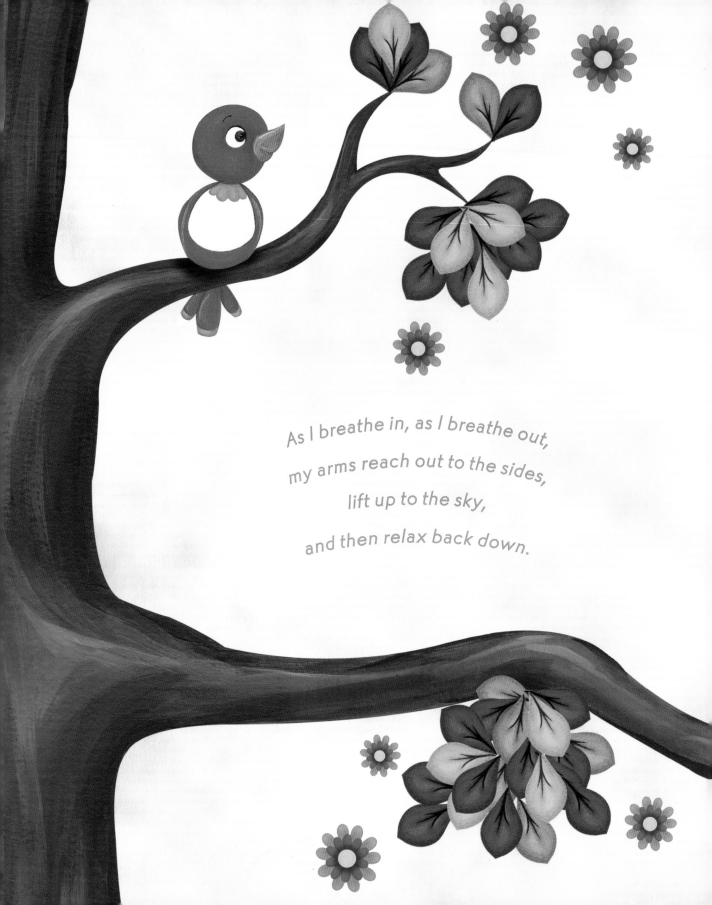

As I breathe in, as I breathe out,

my arms reach out to the sides,

lift up to the sky,

and then relax back down.

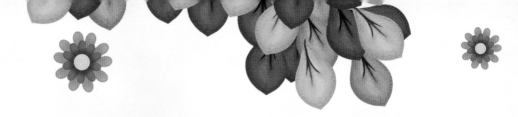

My first breath is long and deep,

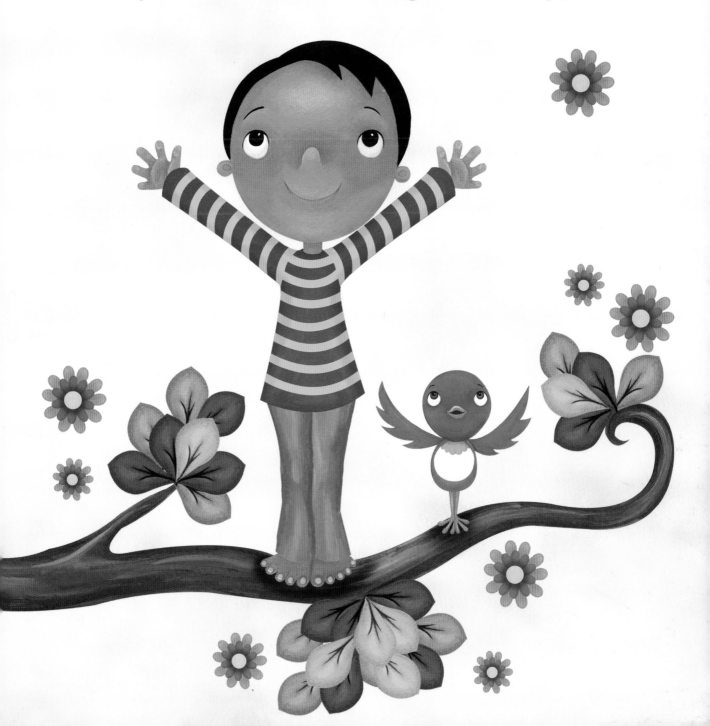

As I breathe in, as I breathe out,
I twist my whole body
from side to side and
swing my arms back and forth.

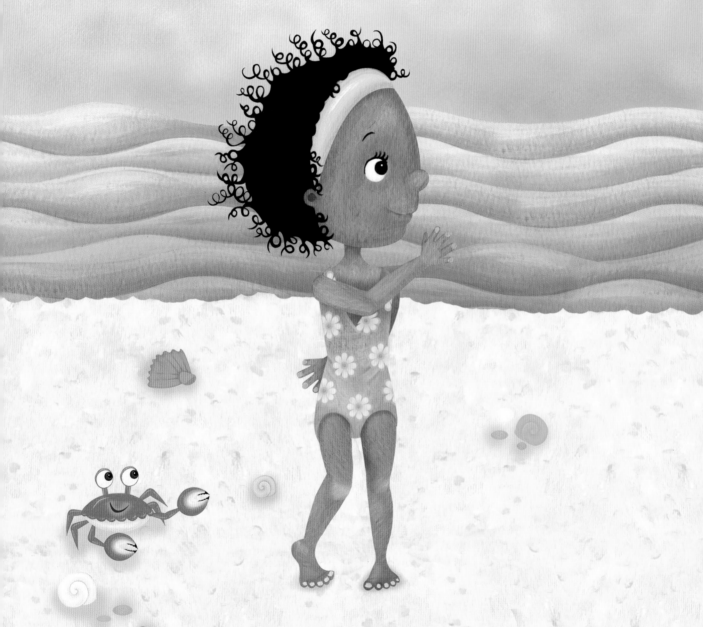

I twist and turn to shake off sleep.

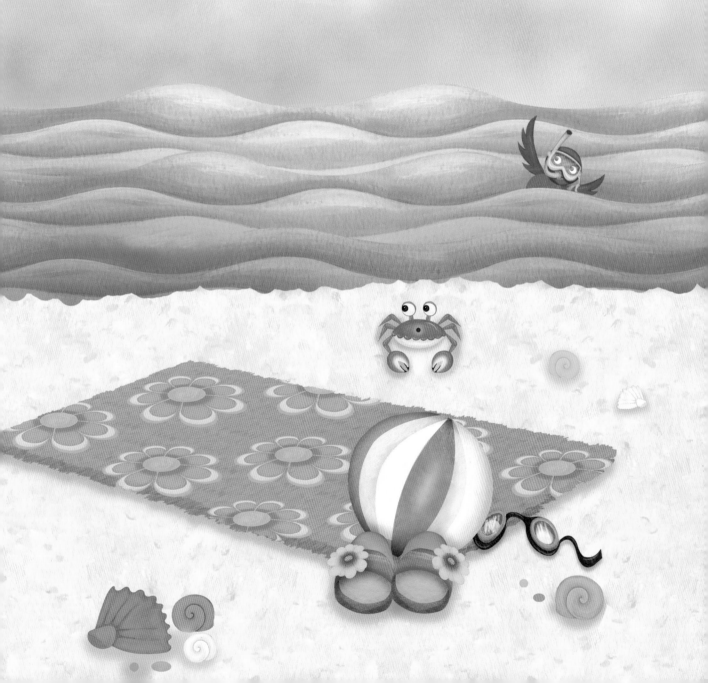

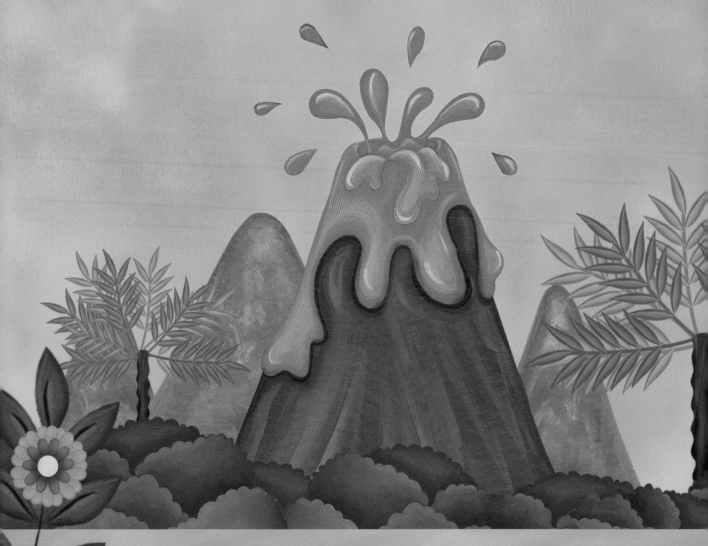

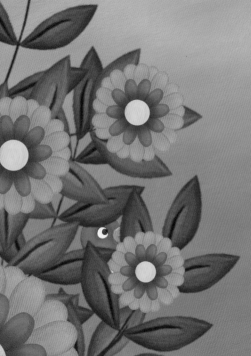

As I breathe in, as I breathe out,
I lift up on tiptoes
and reach my fingers high.

Today I'm a fiery volcano reaching high,

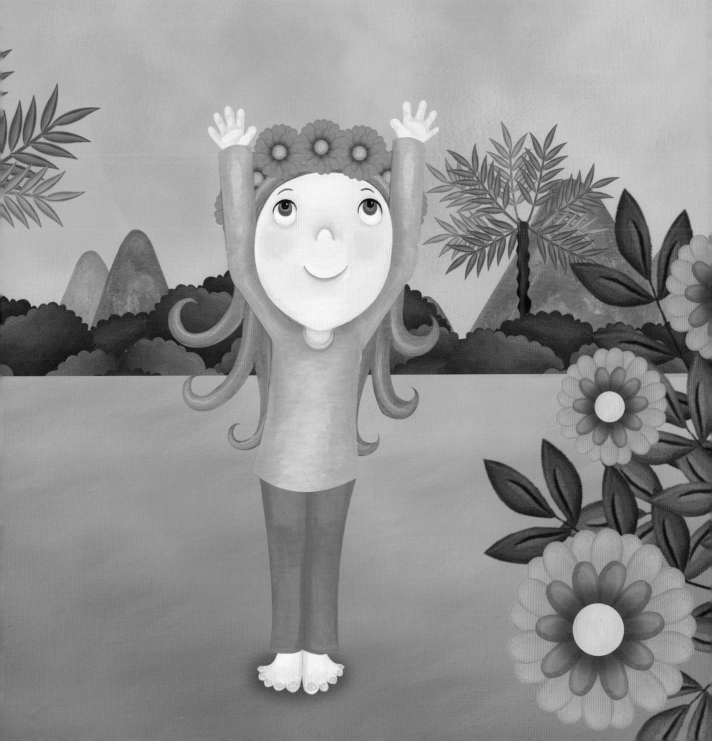

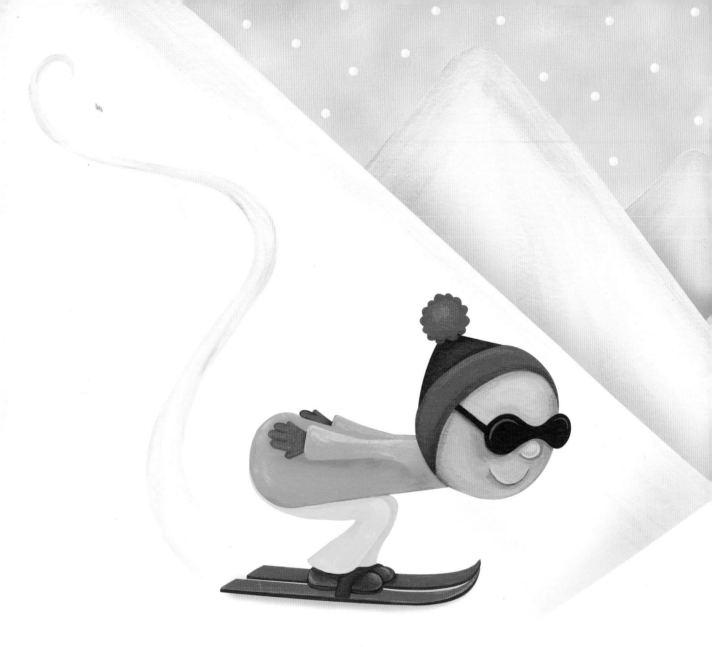

As I breathe in, as I breathe out,

I bend my knees

and sweep my arms back.

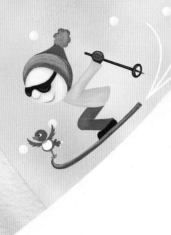

a brave ski jumper ready to fly,

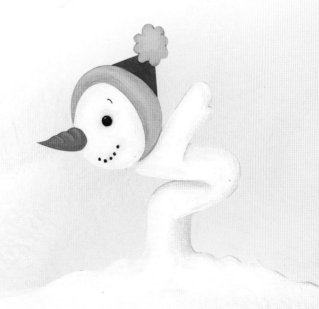

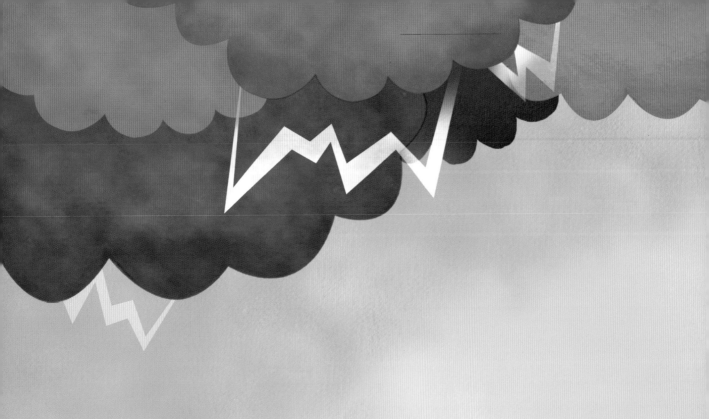

a lightning bolt flashing across the sky.

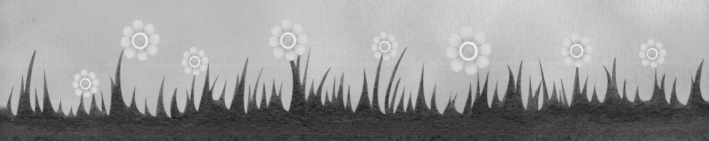

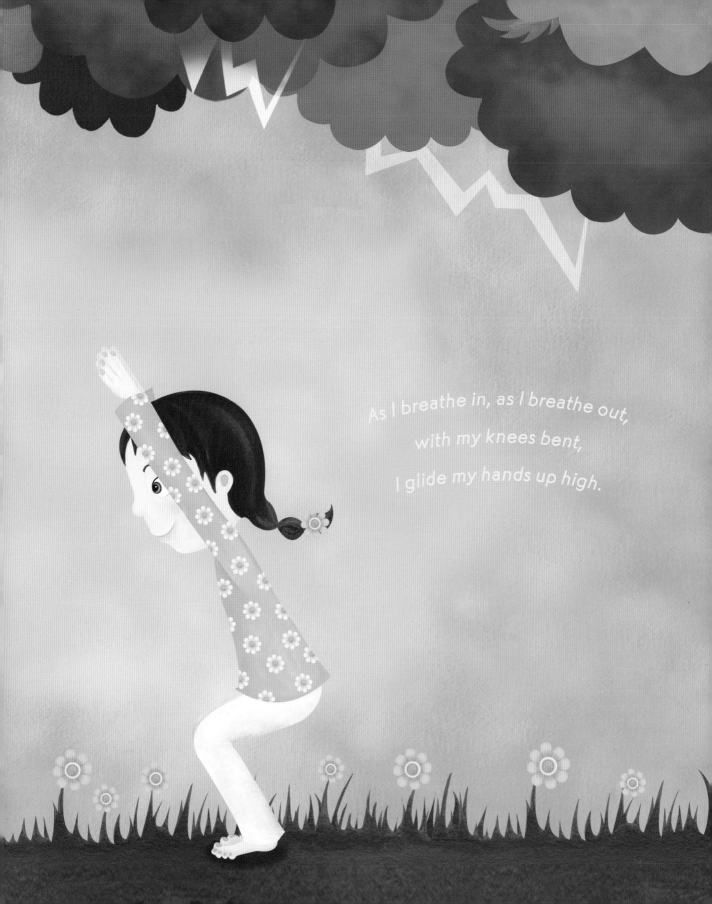

As I breathe in, as I breathe out,
with my knees bent,
I glide my hands up high.

As I breathe in, as I breathe out,
I press down through my feet
and stretch my spine so it is long.
I roll my shoulders back
and press my palms together.

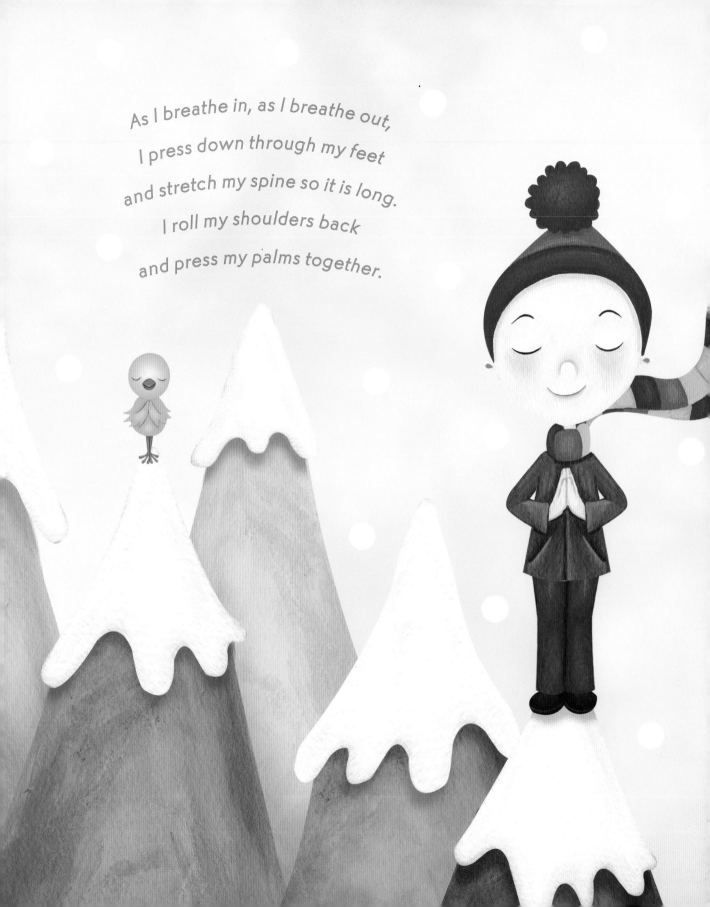

Today I'm also a mountain, quiet and still,

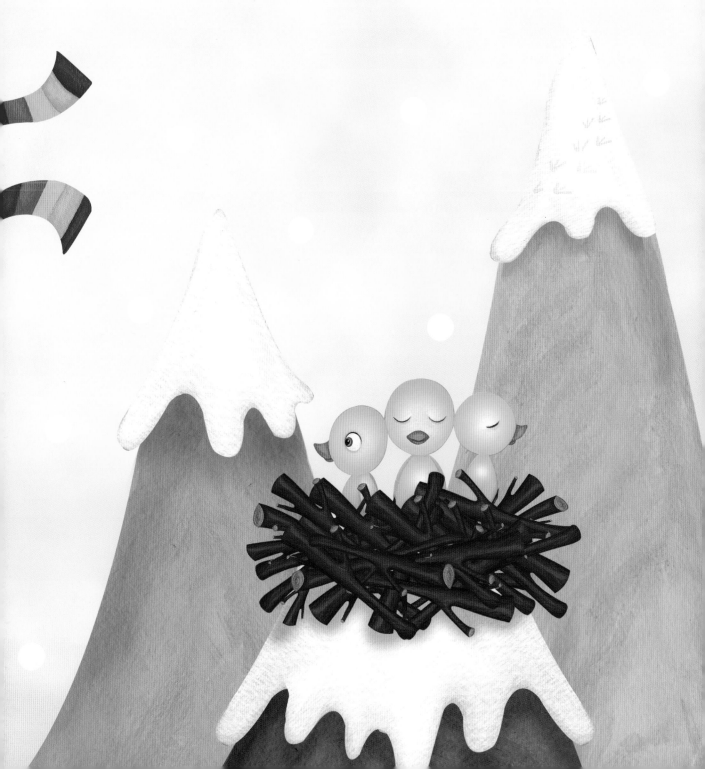

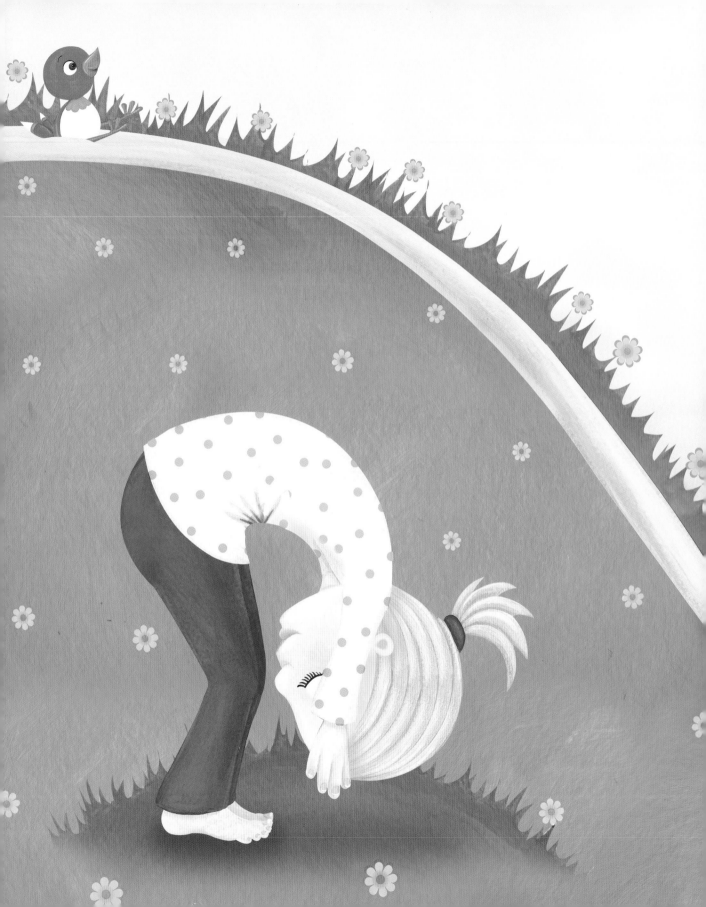

a gentle stream flowing downhill,

As I breathe in, as I breathe out,
I round my back,
bend my knees, and
roll down to the ground.

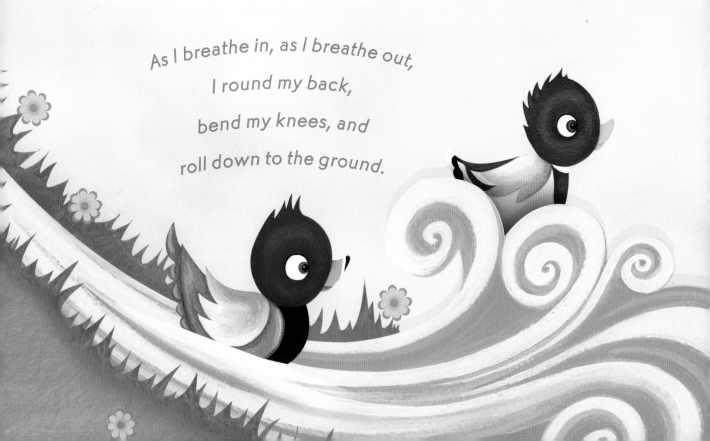

a playful dog stretching with skill.

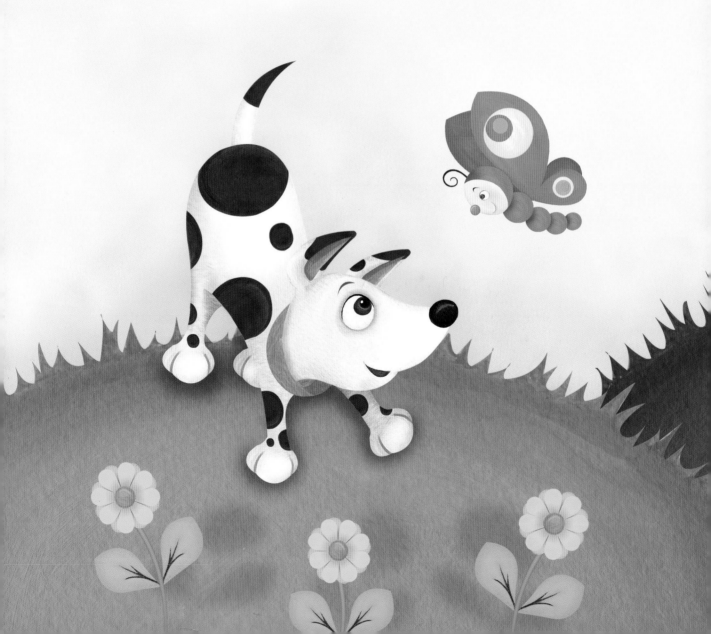

As I breathe in, as I breathe out,

I press my palms and feet

into the earth and

raise my hips up to the sky.

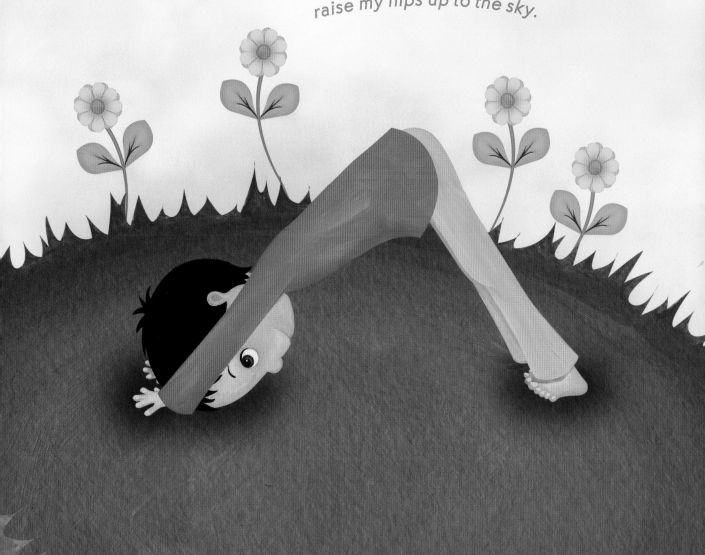

Today I'm an explorer, calm and awake,

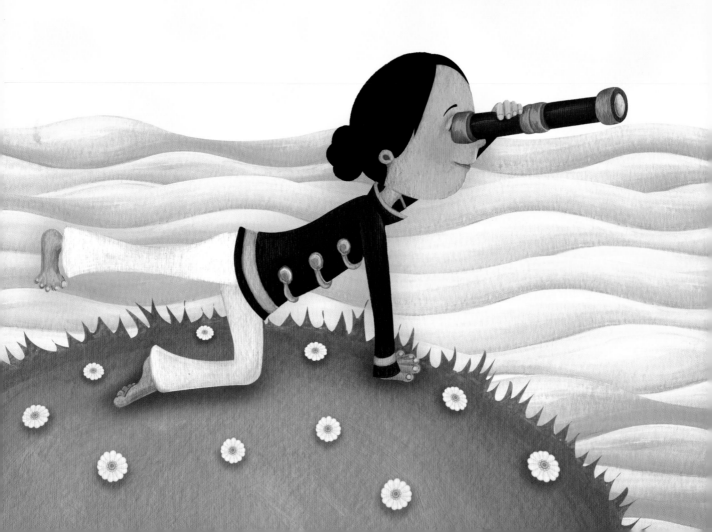

As I breathe in, as I breathe out,

on hands and knees

I bring my left hand forward,

lift my right leg back,

and balance. Then I switch sides.

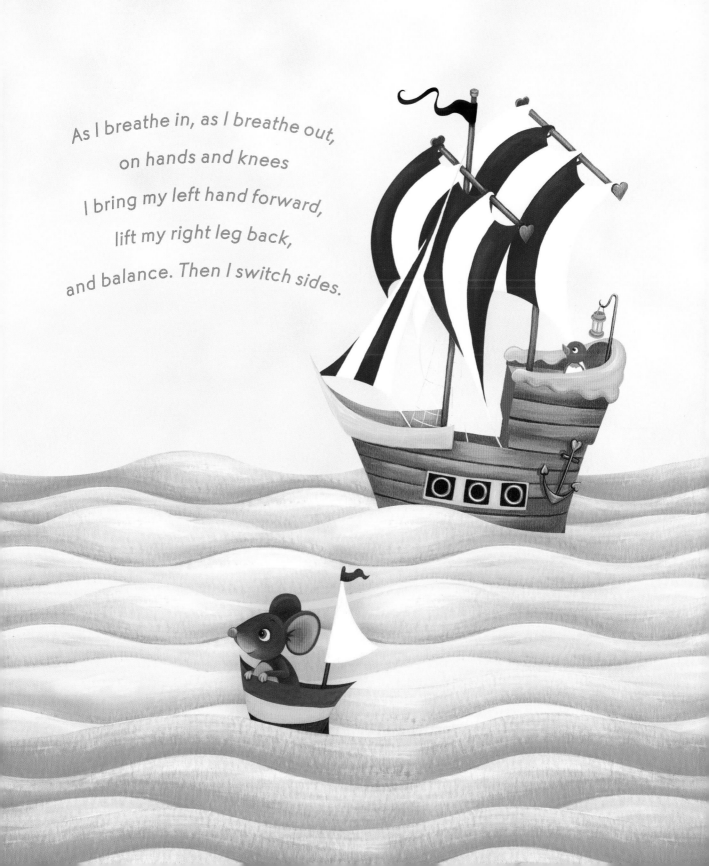

crossing bridges on the paths I take,

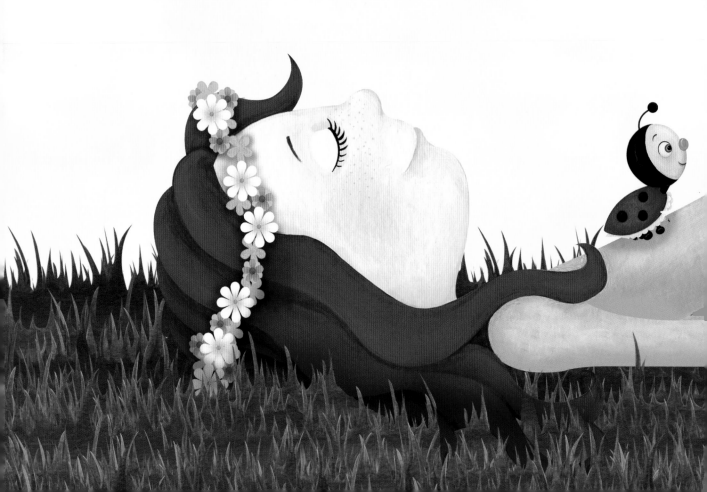

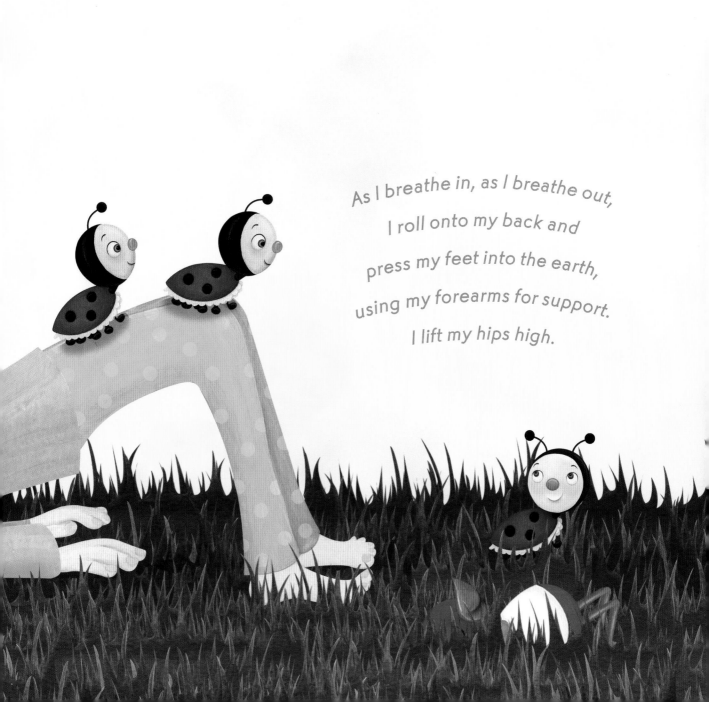

As I breathe in, as I breathe out,
I roll onto my back and
press my feet into the earth,
using my forearms for support.
I lift my hips high.

sailing boats on the journeys I make.

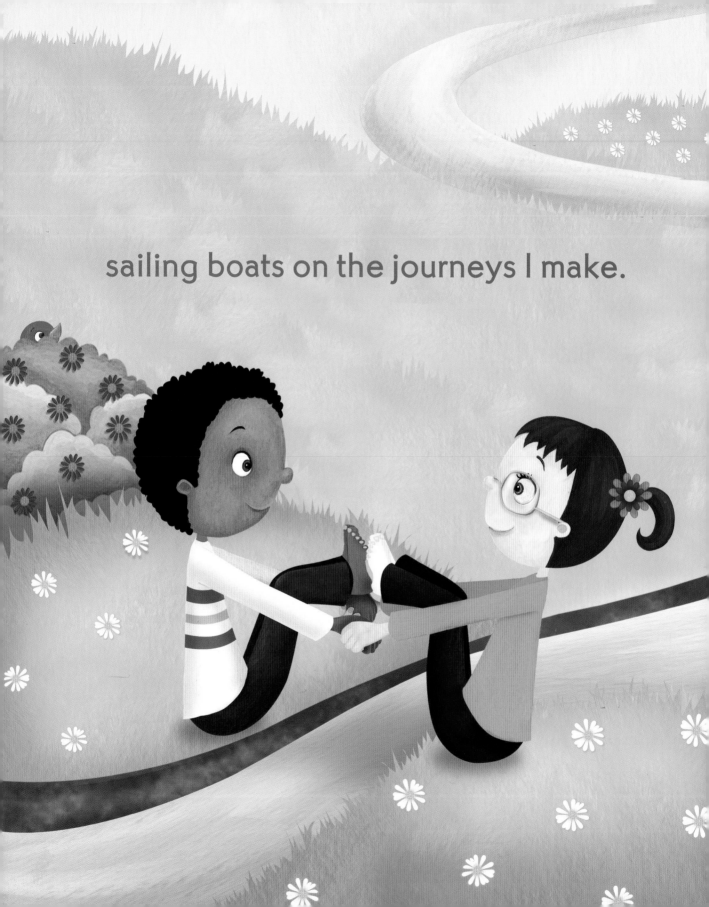

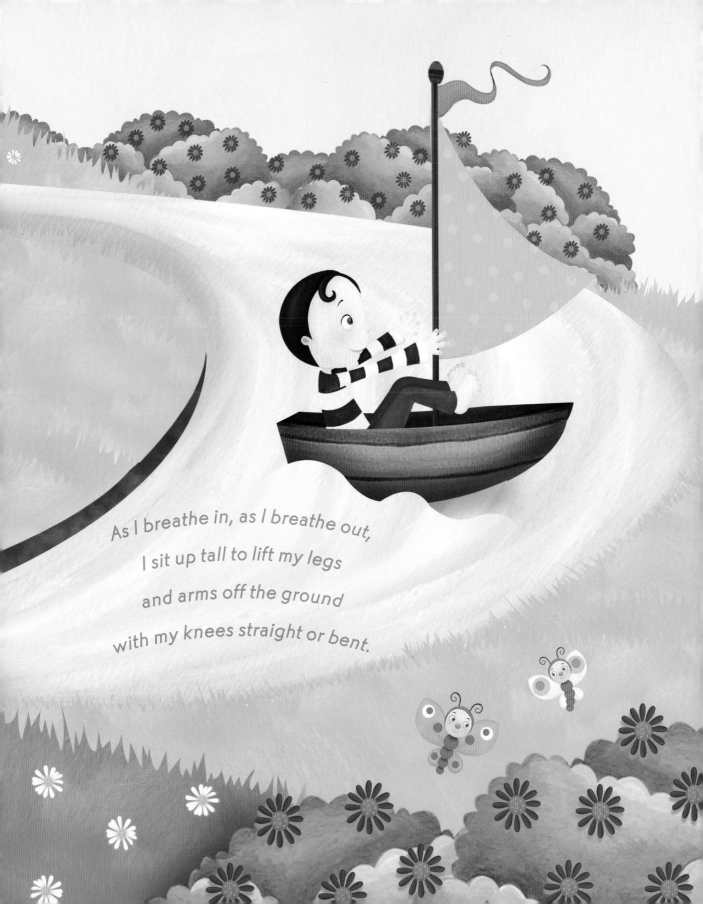

As I breathe in, as I breathe out,
I sit up tall to lift my legs
and arms off the ground
with my knees straight or bent.

Calm and awake, "I can do this!"
is all I need to say.

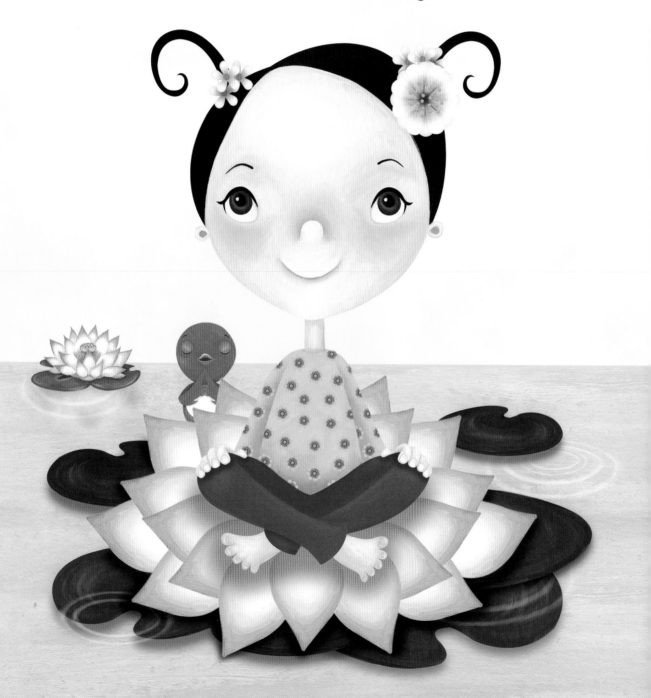

A deep breath in, a long breath out—
I am ready for the day!

As I breathe in, as I breathe out,
I sit with my legs crossed.
My spine grows taller,
my shoulders roll back,
and I rest my hands on my knees.

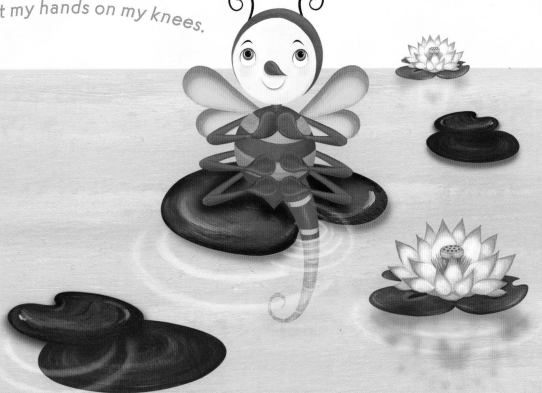

The Good Morning Yoga Flow

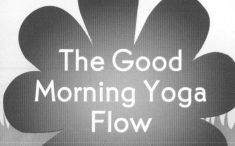

Sun Breath

My arms reach out to the sides, lift up to the sky, and then relax back down.

Tummy Twist

I twist my whole body from side to side and swing my arms back and forth.

Volcano

I lift up on tiptoes and reach my fingers high.

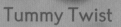
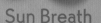

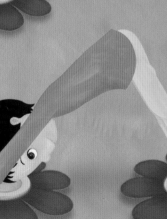

Downward Dog

I press my palms and feet into the earth and raise my hips up to the sky.

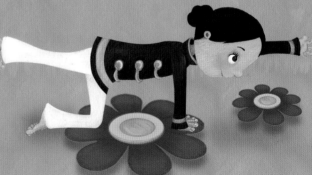

Balancing Table

On hands and knees I bring my left hand forward, lift my right leg back, and balance. Then I switch sides.

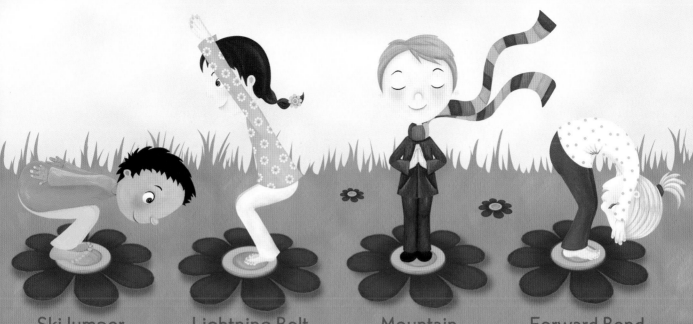

Ski Jumper

I bend my knees and sweep my arms back.

Lightning Bolt

With my knees bent, I glide my hands up high.

Mountain

I press down through my feet and stretch my spine so it is long. I roll my shoulders back and press my palms together.

Forward Bend

I round my back, bend my knees, and roll down to the ground.

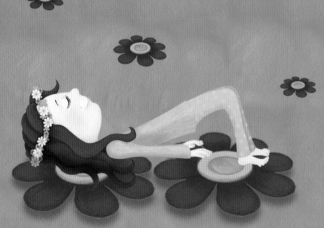

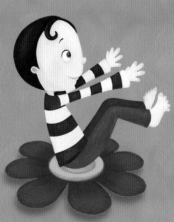

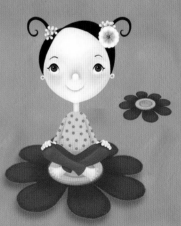

Bridge

I roll onto my back and press my feet into the earth, using my forearms for support. I lift my hips high.

Boat

I sit up tall to lift my legs and arms off the ground with my knees straight or bent.

Awake

I sit with my legs crossed. My spine grows taller, my shoulders roll back, and I rest my hands on my knees.

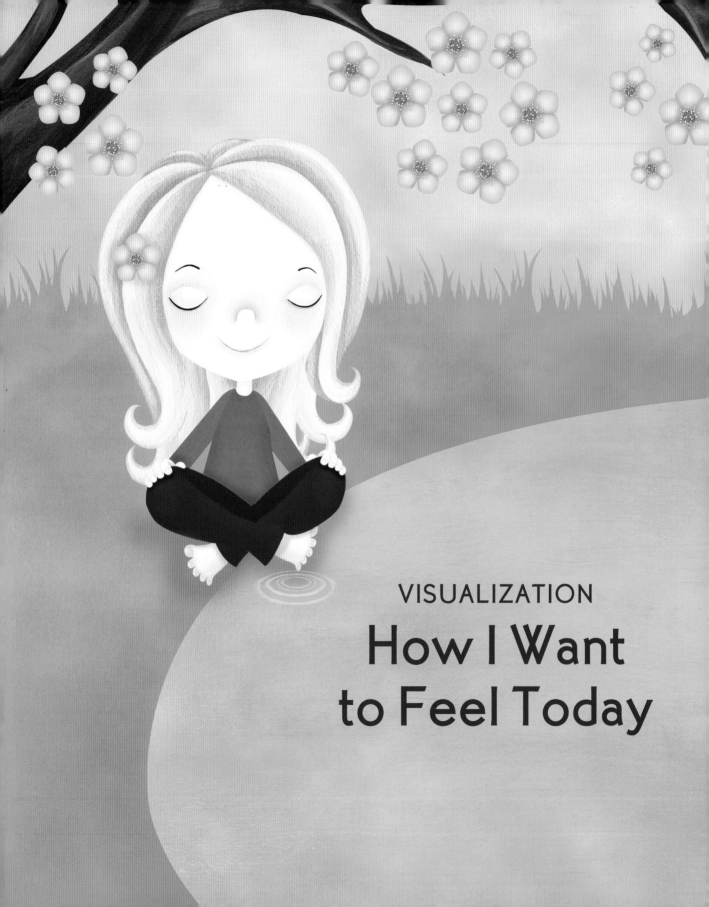

VISUALIZATION

How I Want to Feel Today

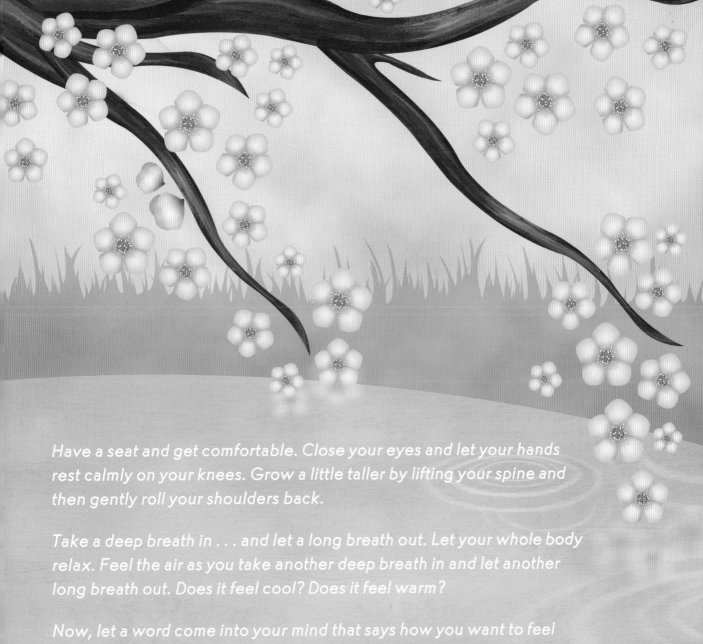

Have a seat and get comfortable. Close your eyes and let your hands rest calmly on your knees. Grow a little taller by lifting your spine and then gently roll your shoulders back.

Take a deep breath in . . . and let a long breath out. Let your whole body relax. Feel the air as you take another deep breath in and let another long breath out. Does it feel cool? Does it feel warm?

Now, let a word come into your mind that says how you want to feel today. It could be a word like joyful, kind, friendly, or curious. It could be a word like happy, peaceful, enthusiastic, or brave. Choose the word that best describes how you want to feel. Hold it in your mind.

As you breathe in, fill yourself up with the feeling you want . . . and as you breathe out, send this feeling out into the world. Feel how you want to be today. Take another deep breath in . . . and let a long breath out. Open your eyes. You are ready for this day.

About Sounds True

Sounds True is a multimedia publisher whose mission is to inspire and support personal transformation and spiritual awakening. Founded in 1985 and located in Boulder, Colorado, we work with many of the leading spiritual teachers, thinkers, healers, and visionary artists of our time. We strive with every title to preserve the essential "living wisdom" of the author or artist. It is our goal to create products that not only provide information to a reader or listener, but that also embody the quality of a wisdom transmission.

For those seeking genuine transformation, Sounds True is your trusted partner. At SoundsTrue.com you will find a wealth of free resources to support your journey, including exclusive weekly audio interviews, free downloads, interactive learning tools, and other special savings on all our titles.

To learn more, please visit SoundsTrue.com/freegifts or call us toll-free at 800-333-9185.

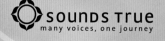

SOUNDS TRUE
many voices, one journey

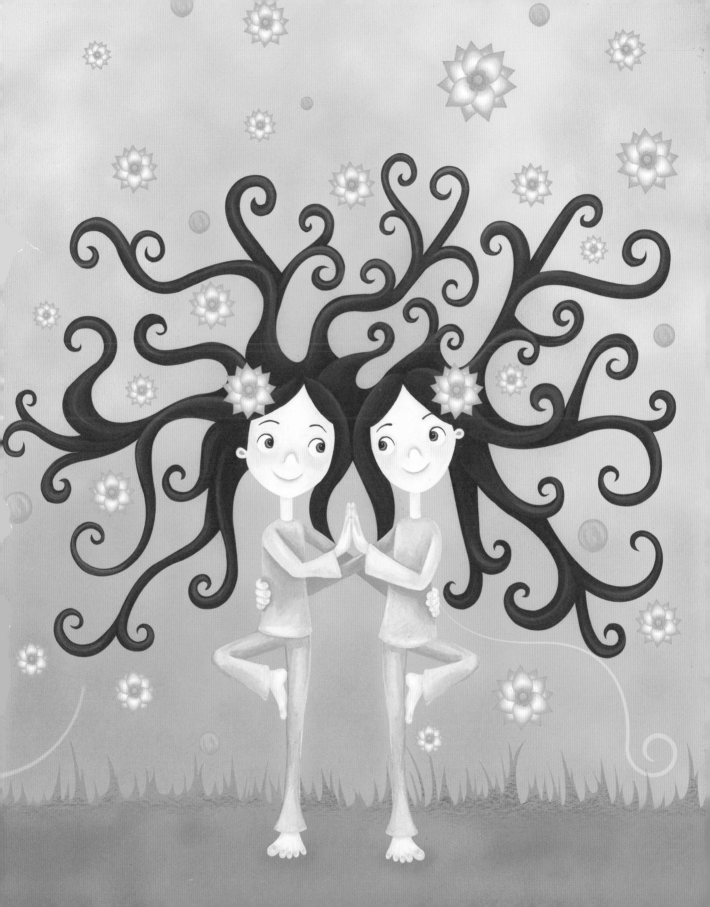

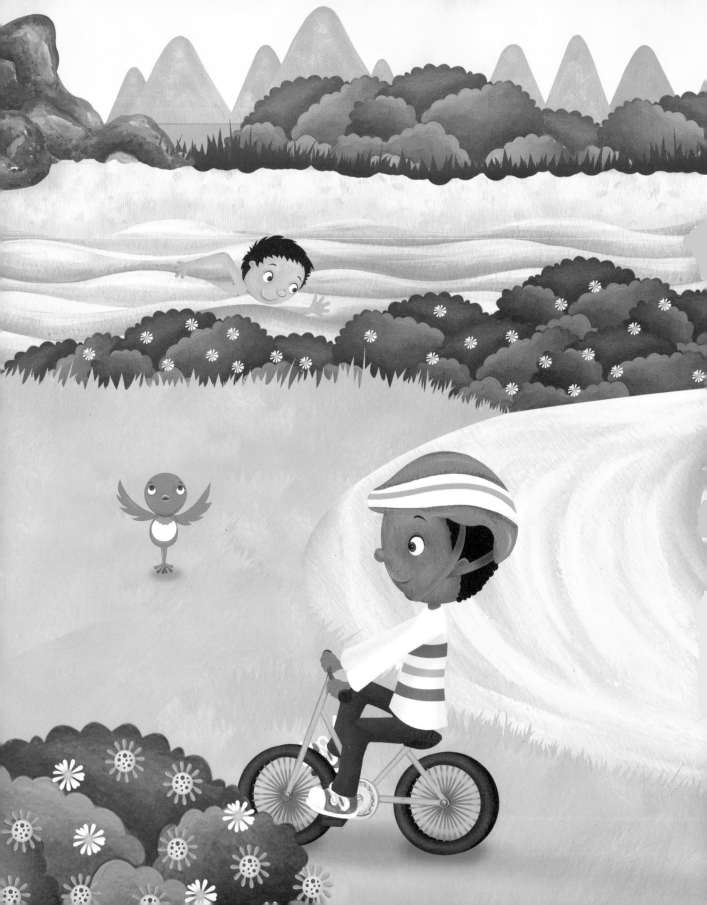